AYURVEDA

Health Tips for Asthma & Allergy Patients

(Methods to Mastering Balance, Well-being and Stress Relief)

Cody Stephens

Published by Knowledge Icons

Cody Stephens

All Rights Reserved

Ayurveda: Health Tips for Asthma & Allergy Patients (Methods to Mastering Balance, Well-being and Stress Relief)

ISBN 978-1-990084-81-2

All rights reserved. No part of this guide may be reproduced in any form without permission in writing from the publisher except in the case of brief quotations embodied in critical articles or reviews.

Legal & Disclaimer

The information contained in this book is not designed to replace or take the place of any form of medicine or professional medical advice. The information in this book has been provided for educational and entertainment purposes only.

The information contained in this book has been compiled from sources deemed reliable, and it is accurate to the best of the Author's knowledge; however, the Author cannot guarantee its accuracy and validity and cannot be held liable for any errors or omissions. Changes are periodically made to this book. You must consult your doctor or get professional medical advice before using any of the suggested remedies, techniques, or information in this book.

Upon using the information contained in this book, you agree to hold harmless the Author from and against any damages, costs, and expenses, including any legal fees potentially resulting from the application of any of the information provided by this guide. This disclaimer applies to any damages or injury caused by the use and application, whether directly or indirectly, of any advice or information presented, whether for breach of contract, tort, negligence, personal injury, criminal intent, or under any other cause of action.

You agree to accept all risks of using the information presented inside this book. You need to consult a professional medical practitioner in order to ensure you are both able and healthy enough to participate in this program.

TABLE OF CONTENTS

INTRODUCTION 1

CHAPTER 1: BASIC PRINCIPLES AND COMPONENTS OF AYURVEDA 6

CHAPTER 2: AYURVEDIC DOSHA 26

CHAPTER 3: LEARN TO SLIM THROUGH AYURVEDA 41

CHAPTER 4: SIX TASTES IN AYURVEDIC DIET 49

CHAPTER 5: AYУГNEdA APPГOACh TO GENITAl HEГPES ... 56

CHAPTER 6: AYURVEDA STRATEGIES TO TREAT VIRAL INFECTIONS AND FEVER 71

CHAPTER 7: FOODS TO EAT FOR YOUR DOSHA 77

CHAPTER 8: AYURVEDA SECRETS FOR PURE ENERGY AND CONTENTMENT 84

CHAPTER 9: BENEFITS OF AYURVEDA DIET AS PER YOUR BODY CONSTITUTION 89

CHAPTER 10: HAIR FALL 93

CHAPTER 11: WHAT IS INSOMNIA? 101

CHAPTER 12: DEMON-RIDDANCE 107

CHAPTER 14: THE CHARACTERISTICS OF KAPHA DOOSHAS ARE –... 113

CHAPTER 15: INCREASING BREAST MILK PRODUCTION: 121

CHAPTER 15: ROOT CAUSE OF SICKNESS 131

CHAPTER 16: ANNAR (POMEGROUND). 138

Introduction

In the past few years we have witnessed a dramatic surge in the popularity of 'Traditional Medicines'. They have strong cultural and historical roots especially among the developing countries like India, Myanmar, etc where the traditional practitioners have commanded great respect over the ages. One such system of Hindu traditional medicine native to Indian subcontinent is Ayurveda. Although it is widely used, there is no scientific evidence for the effectiveness of Ayurvedic medication. The seers of the past, based on their observation and experience, used the natural resources to develop this unique system of medicine which was named as the 'science of life'. Its use basically involves two types of experts – the dispensers and the practitioners. Further the practitioners are divided into two types of therapists – the panchkarma therapists and the Ayurveda dieticians.

Ayurveda is a system encompassing not only science but philosophy and religion as well. Religion here refers to beliefs and disciplines regarding all the aspects of life and one's perception towards them. Philosophy on the other hand denotes love of truth where truth is the source of all life. It is a science of truth. Ayurvedic literature, in essence, is based on the Samkhya philosophy of creation. The science of Ayurveda aims at attaining ideal mental, physical and spiritual health where mental health can be developed by following rules of good conduct; physical health can be attained by following personal hygiene on daily basis; and spiritual well being can be attained by developing a philosophical attitude.

There are 8 branches of Ayurveda –

Medicine - Kaya

Surgery - Shalya

Surgery of head and neck - Ghana

Toxicology – Agada Tantra

Pediatrics - Bala

Psychiatry – Booth Vidya

Sexology - Vajekarana

Geriatic - Rasatyana

Ayurveda and the Human Potential

Ayurveda believes man to be a microcosm i.e. a universe within himself. According to its theory, his individual existence cannot be separated from the overall cosmic manifestation. Thus the Ayurvedic view towards health and disease is a holistic one which takes into account the inherent relationship bw individual and cosmic spirit. Balanced good health depends on the fulfillment of four biological and spiritual instincts - religious, pro-active, financial and the instinct towards freedom. Through the teachings of Ayurveda, the practical knowledge and training of self healing can be acquired by anyone.

Ayurveda and the Western Thought

Western concept of medication tends to generalize for a group of individuals after categorizing them. For e.g. according to western thought, what is common for a number of people constitutes a norm. On the other hand, ayurveda states that norms must be individual specific as every human being manifests a particular temperament and physiology. Ayurveda relies on acceptance, observation, and experience while the western concept revolves around questioning, analysis, and logical deduction. West propounds objectivity while ayurveda champions subjectivity. Due to this difference in approach towards medical concepts, ayurveda is found difficult to comprehend by some western practitioners.

Due to some of the ambiguities as mentioned above, the reader may find some concepts unacceptable by way of logic and reasoning. Hence you are advised to accept the statements and arguments as given in the first reading before your actually attain mastery to question the details. Even in western concept of medicine, some theories are proven to work without fully understanding the reasons behind their working.

Chapter 1: Basic Principles And Components Of Ayurveda

Ayurveda can be translated as "knowledge of life" and it's understandable why. It comes down to a whole life philosophy after all! The key to grasping the nature of Ayurvedic wisdom is perceiving the way everything is interconnected: our energy fields, our physical health, our emotional well-being, our spiritual outlook, our daily habits and routines and so on. If one of these dimensions that make up our personality is ignored, chances are the overall purpose of improving health and maintaining it can be undermined.

What You Should Know about Doshas

The foundation of Ayurvedic philosophy is the idea that universal life force manifests in our physical and mental bodies as three types of energy known as doshas. These bodily humors combine in various proportions in our body in order to shape our individual energetic and metabolic profile according to which we should modify our diet and lifestyle so as to be as healthy as possible. The three doshas are Vata, Pitta, and Kapha. There are various subcategories in each main type of humor. However, for starters, it is enough if we understand what each dosha means. The bottom line is that doshas are energies that run through our body. We sometimes have a combination of these "life forces" – most of us have one or two basic doshas in their makeup. As long as these forces are balanced, we are safe and healthy. However when there's some deregulation in the way our energies intermingle (for instance, if one dosha totally engulfs our physical and mental space), our health suffers and we should take the right steps to brings things back to a state of balance.

Vata dosha

Vata relates mainly to the nervous system. It is associated with a windy quality and in the body it is responsible for imbalances such as flatulence, gout, rheumatism etc. People whose bodies have a preponderance of Vata tend to be thin and rather lanky. The good aspects of this dosha are a high level or mental and physical activity. Vata types are creative and sociable. They love people and traveling and they need to be "in motion" somehow, whether through interpersonal relationships, or by means of their professional and leisure activities.

In a state of perfect balance, Vata types are flexible, imaginative, outgoing, dynamic, and lively. They like to stay mentally stimulated and they are often quite original thinkers. If Vata people are imbalanced, they can get overexcited, anxious, "airy" (think "head-in-the-clouds behavior), overrun by excessive nervous energy, ungrounded etc. An unbalanced Vita can seem unreliable and flaky about promises and commitments they make. A high form of mobility, but also changeability makes it hard for them to stick to routines. Completing projects they start becomes more and more difficult. One could say Vata energy run out of balance looks a bit like ADHD.

People influenced by this dosha enjoy warm and humid weather and don't tolerate winter and cold very well. Vata, when it's out of order, engenders joint problems, cold hands and feet, dry skin, constipation, and nervous disorders. Since Vata can be associated with the windair element, people who are "ruled" by this force have high energy and like staying active and getting in touch with people, but their mood, work performance, and appetite can fluctuate drastically. That's why Vata types sometimes experience sleep and eating disorders. Instead of being constant in their routines, they can jump from one type of food to another while lacking balance and moderation. They can mix food in unhealthy ways and they either sleep too little, or too much. They also often resort to sedatives and stimulants. Insomnia is a rather frequent problem that comes up in the lives of Vata types and so may experience unhealthy eating patterns (such as eating too much at once or going without food for too many hours, likely only on coffee or other pseudo-energizers).

Pitta dosha

While Vata can be partly associated with the sanguine temperament, **Pitta** energy has to do with the yellow bile and in the Hippocratic system, it corresponds to the choleric energy. Although there is no fixed and absolute connection between Ayurvedic perspective on bodily humors and Hippocrates's theory of temperaments, one cannot help noticing certain similarities between the two systems of human personality, behavior, and health. Pitta is thus the bilious humor secreted in the area between the stomach and the bowels, flowing through the liver and reaching our spleen, eyes, heart, and skin. Energetically Pitta has a "fiery" quality and its movement through the body evokes heat. This energy principle uses bile to direct and regulate metabolism and is connected mainly with the digestive system as a focal area of activity.

Pitta types are ruled by the fire element. Temperamentally they are energetic, highly excitable, strong, intense, and irritable. Physically they tend to have medium to strong build, high endurance and quite powerful musculature. However their endurance seems to have an energetic basis more often than not. The overall impression is that it's not their physical body that is a main source of force for them, but rather a center of mental and metabolic energy that makes them fiery, slightly aggressive, and feisty. They sometimes have freckled skin that easily becomes reddish in the sun or during exercisemassage. Pitta folks are quite strong-willed and stubborn and they know how to stay on their chosen track, especially since they can quite objectively evaluate their own abilities and they know what they are good at. Pitta people can come across as slightly arrogant if they know they are right or the best at doing something.

Since they are not the most diplomatic of the doshas, they may be a bit abrupt and harsh with other people sometimes, especially when they get impatient to get the job done and they see others are messing with the efficiency of a project or proving to be incompetent. Pitta people approach work with highly contaminating energy if they collaborate with the right people.

Overall their personality stands out through intensity and competitiveness. These people are natural leaders, ambitious go-getters, proficient professionals, and quick learners in almost everything they do. Pitta implies high mental energy and a drive towards activity and positive change (think "getting things done" and "making the world a better place" in one and the same person). Pitta folks have an exceptional ability to comprehend and master new skills, fields of study, theories, and concepts.

Since they usually have high standards and are so quick to learn new things and assimilate them into their practical know-how, Pitta people can seem impatient, judgmental, or intolerant towards people they see as inefficient, slower, less driven, or less focused than themselves. Since they are usually high achievers who cannot stand passivity, inertia, and general stagnation, it's quite understandable that Pitta folks may have a hard time when dealing with people who take things more easily and casually than themselves. Or it's actually other people who have a harder time in the presence of Pitta folks more often than not. Why? It's mainly because Pitta energy implies less people skills and more work efficiency, vision, and drive to succeed and overcome obstacleschallenges.

Thus, a Pitta person can come across as abrupt and harsh when they deal with someone who moves too slowly or makes many mistakes. They are usually quite resistant when criticized – it's the others who may "suffer" because of the fiery nature of the Pitta person.

Pitta implies strong digestion and intense appetites. People ruled by this dosha often carve food and they can show the same intensity in relationships or in front of challenges. They may get bored and feel restless if too little is demanded from them. Their most suitable professions and lifestyles are fast-paced, high-standard, and competence-oriented. If a Pitta person missesskips a meal, they are likely to become grumpy and irritable, even looking for fights and taking it out on others instead.

When imbalanced, Pitta is usually associated with health conditions such as inflammation, digestive problems, rashes, excessive anger, acne, and loose stool. In order to stay healthy, Pitta people need to manage their "fire" and channel their high drive and energy in productive activities. When set on getting something done or improving things, a Pitta person can move mountains. However when out of balance, the choleric energy of a Pitta person can risk becoming destructive.

Kapha dosha

Kapha is associated with "liquid" energy and it relates to bodily fluids, mucus, lubrication etc. As such, this life force ensures that nutrients are carried throughout the body and maintains a good circulation of fluid in our organs. People who are influenced by this humor have strong frames and can stay fit and athletic, provided that they exercise regularly. Otherwise the Kapha energy that rules their personality can give them a tendency to gain weight.

Although this life force is mainly associated with the water element, one can also see traces of "earth" matter as a principle that gives consistency and solidity. Kapha types are stable, hardworking, compassionate, and loyal. They usually like doing things in a methodical way which may seem a bit slow to some people (especially to Pitta folks), but the Kapha person is actually only approaching an issue in a step-by-step manner. Kapha people get things done, but they like keeping their own pace. They move slowly, but surely towards their goals. That said, their tendency towards stability makes them prefer predictable routines in their personal and professional lives.

However not everything is so positive when dealing with a Kapha type. As we've already seen when discussing other life forces, imbalance can seriously undermine the advantages of a humor in one's personality. When Kapha is imbalanced in the body, people ruled by this principle can become too rigid, unmotivated, excessively stubborn, set in their ways, stuck in a rut, and complacent with routines even if change is imperative. Kapha people have slow metabolism and their appetite for both food and stimulation is healthy, but less intense than in the other two types. In order to escape monotony and stagnation, Kapha types should allow themselves to move to new environments, meet new people, and seek new experiences. So as to stay fit and keep their metabolism in an optimal state, Kapha folks should occasionally practice fasting as a diet or as a means of regulating their digestion and health.

Your Doshic Constitution

Now you are probably asking yourself if only one dosha is predominant in our bodies. Some people are primarily influenced by one life force and it's quite visible in their life that one dosha predominates. By that, I mean the overall temperament, preferences, or health problems that they have to face. This condition is nevertheless not exactly ideal, since too much of one single dosha in one's personality and body can be a sign of imbalance. When one dosha has all the power over the body, people often display negative sides of their dosha (e.g extreme stubbornness, too much anger, impaired capacity to focus etc). That's why it's optimal when one main dosha is nevertheless counteracted (and balanced) by the presence and activity of a second (and even a third one). When two or three doshas work in unison in a harmonious proportion, the body and the mind are balanced and most likely quite healthy.

The Two-doshic Types

Most people are ruled by two doshas. Thus, they share some of the qualities that are usually associated with two distinct doshas. Of course it would be too contradictory and almost unbelievable to have all traits associated with a dosha manifest themselves. How could one be competitive, challenging, fast-paced, and easily angered the Pitta style and methodical, stable, compassionate, and slow at the same time? However, quite often several characteristics of two different doshas converge in the makeup of one's personality. Thus, they regulate themselves and engender a beneficial balance.

Sometimes people who have a dual constitution may experience a form of split or dilemma. For instance, in certain situations, one dosha will predominate and under other circumstances the other dosha will have the upper hand. As long as the right dosha dictates in the right context, that's not necessarily a disadvantage. For instance, it's great if you can be efficient, focused, and fast at work while being loyal, tactful, kind, and consistent with friends and family.

Ayurveda teaches us that the best way to manage a dual constitution is to mind seasonal cycles. For example, if you have a vata-pitta or vata-kapha constitution, during autumn (a vata season in Ayurvedic books), you can balance your body and mind by following a regimen that decreases the corresponding life force. This regimen includes diet, exercise, and other routines that should shape your lifestyle during that interval. During summer or spring, you'd have to follow a pitta-decreasing regimen.

What Does Being Tri-doshic Imply?

Some people are tri-doshic, which means they have equal amounts of each energylife force. Such a person is the epitome or balance and power; however you should know this combination is quite rare. A tri-doshic person can be very strong, multifaceted, stable, versatile, complex, and positive when the energies are in balance. If they are out of balance, the person may find themselves "torn" between tendencies and drives that derive from different doshas and they can experience poor health.

One of the basic principles of Ayurveda implies achieving balance by noticing potential imbalances in your mind and body. Such imbalances may be inborn or they may arise from your environment, your diet, your emotional state, or your life experiences. The key is learning to include in your life practices that will counterbalance any negative influence of a dosha. Once again, if you are a tri-doshic person, you should maintain balance by means of paying attention to seasonal principles and adjusting your diet and lifestyle accordingly. For example, in autumn a tri-doshic person should encourage their vata constitution and follow a vata-balancing regimen. Similarly, you can nourish your optimal energy when the season is right. You should adopt a pitta-balancing lifestyle when the weather is hot and a kapha-balancing regimen during cold and damp seasons.

Chapter 2: Ayurvedic Dosha

The Three Types of Dosha

Have you ever considered why people can be so different in temperament and behavior? Why are some individuals hyperactive and quick-moving, while others exude calm and peace? Why can some individuals eat a five-course dinner with little effort, while others can scarcely complete a plate of mixed greens? Why are some people characteristically happy, while others carry the weight of the world on their shoulders? Modern genetic studies have offered some insights, yet they don't explain all of the nuances that make us so different from one another. Ayurveda addresses this with the Three Doshas: Vata, Pitta and Kapha.

The Doshas are natural energies found throughout the human body and psyche. They represent all physical and mental processes and furnish each living being with an individual outline for wellbeing and satisfaction.

The Doshas draw from the Five Elements and their related properties. Vata is comprised of Space and Air, Pitta of Fire and Water, and Kapha of Earth and Water.

If you are a man with a predominately Vata constitution you will have physical and mental qualities that mirror the basic characteristics of Space and Air. That is the reason you are quick-thinking, thin, and fast-moving. If you are a Pitta type, then you will exhibit qualities of Fire and Water, for example, a passionate nature, be slightly impatient and prone to freckling and burning. If you are a Kapha type, you will most often have a strong, sturdy body and a cool personality, mirroring the basic components of Earth and Water. While one Dosha prevails in many people, a second Dosha normally is at work as well. This is known as a "double doshic constitution".

VATA

Vata dominates all functions of the brain and body. It controls blood stream, disposal of toxins, breathing and the development of the psyche. The primary areas of Vata in the body are the colon, thighs, bones, joints, ears, skin, cerebrum, and nerve tissues. Physiologically, Vata involves all bodily processes, for example, breathing, talking, nervous system tasks, cellular regeneration in the muscles and tissues, digestion, waste disposal, and a woman's menstrual cycle. Mentally, Vata involves our ability to communicate, imagine, adapt, and the speed with which we process information.

The well-adjusted Vata individual is dynamic, innovative, and gifted with a characteristic capacity to express themselves and convey thought. When out of balance, a Vata type can be like a storm, negative qualities rapidly dominating the positive characteristics. Basic indications of Vata imbalance include nervousness and physically manifestations like as dry skin.

What you need to do to balance your Vata Dosha.

Eat a Vata supporting diet.

Eat in a serene environment.

Engage in wholesome and thoughtful exercises (like investing energy in nature).

Follow a routine.

Go to bed early.

Meditate every day.

Do gentle physical activity like yoga, swimming, kendo, or walking.

What you need to avoid to prevent imbalance of your Vata Dosha.

Eating Vata draining foods.

Eating while on edge or depressed.

Eating on the run.

Drinking alcohol, espresso or dark tea (anything high in caffeine).

Smoking cigarettes.

Maintaining a hectic, unpredictable schedule.

Going to bed late.

PITTA

Pitta is responsible for the body's metabolism digestive system and energy levels. It entails the body's natural acids, hormones, chemicals, and bile. While Pitta is most identified with the component of Fire, it is the fluidity of these substances that accounts for the component of Water in Pitta's make-up.

The principle areas of Pitta in the body are the small intestine, stomach, liver, spleen, pancreas, blood, eyes, and sweat glands. Physiologically, Pitta gives the body warmth and vitality. It represents all procedures identified with transformation in the brain and body. Mentally, Pitta oversees happiness, strength, self-discipline, indignation, envy, and mental observation. It likewise gives the brilliant light of the mind.

For example, when an individual is said to be "overheated", an over-abundance of Pitta is generally the cause. Like a small campfire may transform into an out-of-control forest fire if not properly tended, the internal flame of the brain and body must be held within proper levels.

Once you have familiarized yourself with what your Dosha is, you will better understand why you are the way you are and be better-equipped to heal yourself. You will be able to attain contentment and good health.

What you need to do to balance your Pitta Dosha.

The most important words to remember: cool, calm, moderation.

Eat a Pitta supporting diet.

Eat in a calm setting.

Avoid synthetic stimulants.

Engage in calming exercises (in nature).

Meditate every day.

Do gentle physical activity, for example, yoga, swimming, judo, or walking.

What you need to avoid to prevent imbalance of your Pitta Dosha

Eating Pitta draining foods.

Eating when angry.

Drinking espresso, dark tea or alcohol.

Smoking cigarettes.

Setting unreasonable expectations.

Being excessively aggressive.

KAPHA

Kapha represents Earth and Water and is defined as "that which sticks". It is the foundation that gives the body physical frame, structure, and ensures the smooth working of every one of its parts. Kapha can be considered the fundamental bond, glue, and grease of the body all in one.

The characteristics of Kapha are a heavier build that tends to easily become overweight, slower on the uptake but retain information well, and slow-paced. A Kapha individual will demonstrate similar physical and mental qualities whether in an adjusted and imbalanced state.

The principle areas of Kapha in the body are the midsection, throat, lungs, head, lymph, soft tissue, connective tissue, ligaments, and tendons. Physiologically, Kapha is responsible for supplying nourishment to our tissues, allows for ease of movement in our joints, stores vitality, and identifies with bodily fluids, for example, mucous and lymph. Mentally, Kapha oversees love, persistence, forgiveness, greed, connection, and mental idleness. Kapha grounds Vata and Pitta and helps balance the awkward nature identified with those Doshas.

You are a kapha if you sometimes try to be the center of a conversation or a party but no matter how hard you try you just can't attract the attention the room. Do you ever feel like you are too delicate and fragile for the world? Don't worry, this is just your Dosha, your constitution.

What you need to do to balance your Kapha Dosha

Eat a Kapha supporting diet.

Eat in familiar, comfortable area.

Avoid an over-indulgent way of life.

Focus on down-time daily.

Ensure your lifestyle is orderly and your home clean.

Make time for reflective exercises, like composing.

Ensure you are not taken for granted.

Go to bed early and rise ahead of schedule, with no daytime naps.

What you need to avoid to prevent imbalance of your Kapha Dosha

Eating Kapha draining foods.

Overeating.

Eating your feelings (trying to fill an emotional void with food).

Spending a lot of time in cool, damp environments.

Avoiding physical activity and instead spending too much time watching TV, etc.

Avoiding learning difficulties.

Dosha: How you can determine it

There are many quizzes that help you determine your body type (prakriti) or Dosha.

The purpose of such tests is to discern your body-type as it is denoted by the three types above. Check out the following links to take one of these tests:

http:www.whatsyourDosha.comquiz

http:www.Doshaguru.comDoshaquiz

One of the main questions asked is the type of skin you have. So you'll need to choose from dry and rough, thin and sensitive, or thick and oily. Also asked is how your eyes look and feel. Are they small and dry or wide and teary? The temperature of your body is also crucial to the categorization.

Although the tests include many physical descriptions, a crucial thing to know is the way you act when under pressure: anxious, forceful or discouraged? You additionally need to note your sleep habits: light sleeper, sound sleeper or deep sleeper? What sort of climate do you favor: chilly, hot or wet? It is likewise vital to know whether you get in shape effortlessly or have trouble improving your physique. Your hunger and dietary patterns are noted, as well as your bowel habits: are you prone to constipation or loose stools? Finally, your temperament is asked: easy-going or easily-excited?

Ayurveda takes everything into consideration when determining your body type. Is it accurate to say that you are irritable or not? Do you have a great memory or not? Do you accomplish things on time or not? Do you have frail joints?

Answer the questions based on how you have been the majority of your life. For instance, on the off-chance that you have been thin the greater part of your life but recently put on a great deal of weight, then reply as it applies to your normal body type. In the event that you have just fallen ill, then answer in view of how you were before the disease.

Keep in mind to answer in light of what is and not on what you need to be. In the event that you are experiencing issues with a few questions, then ask a companion or relative to help you. They should be able to give you a fair assessment.

Remember, Vata is you, Pitta is you and Kapha is you. All these traits and qualities reside within you. And once you are able to relate with your appropriate Dosha, you will know how to conquer it, feed it and work with it according to your own wants and needs.

Chapter 3: Learn To Slim Through

Ayurveda

Our prehistoric ancestors lived during times of alternating food bounty and scarcity. They needed an efficient way to store fuel for the slim times. When nutrition was abundant, their bodies adapted by storing fat. In times of severe deprivation, they dieted which was not by choice. This survival adaptation is still with us today. When you diet, cutting your caloric intake, you are signaling to your body that you are in the slim times. Your metabolism slows and you start storing fat. As everyone knows, you will eventually lose weight with this deprivation. The problem is that you will lose not only the unwanted fat, but also vital slim body mass.

The leading theory in metabolic weight control today involves the boosting of food burning to use up excess calories through body heat. Many leading herbs for weight loss work in this way. One such herb is green tea. Several pungent Ayurvedic herbs, including cayenne and ginger, have been demonstrated to promote thermogenesis. Garlic also assists in burning fat through increasing metabolism.

An Ayurvedic resin, called guggul, is a standby medicine for the management of body fats. Particularly valuable in lowering cholesterol, guggul rivals any other natural substance. Without dietary adjustments, guggul has lowered total cholesterol by over 20%, while increasing good HDL cholesterol by more than 30%.

The most well known herbal formula in Ayurveda is triphala (three fruits). Containing amla (Emblica officinalis), bibitaki (Terminalia belerica), and haritaki (Terminalia chebula), it has a light laxative effect and is well studied as a supreme general detoxifier and antioxidant.

The combination of guggul and triphala has showed a surprising effect in controlling body fat.

The name of the famous Asian herb, Gurmar, means killer of sweet. Gurmar (Gymnema sylvestre) is an extensively studied and widely used herb in the treatment of diabetes, which of course is closely related to long term obesity.

Gurmar has been proven in study after study to increase the production and activity of insulin produced in the body. This insulin increase is thought by many experts to be the primary successful method of promoting fat burning. Gurmar is extremely safe, with no known side effects. Through these, ayurveda gives us an ideal herb for treating the diabetic obesity.

Fiber is critical to many functions in the intestinal tract, including digestion and waste elimination. It also has a mild cholesterol lowering effect. Many new studies propose that water-soluble fibers may also help individuals lose weight. Taken with a meal, they produce a feeling of fullness. The other anti-fat benefits of fiber include reducing the absorption of total calories, promoting blood sugar control and enhancing the effects of insulin. Dietary fiber is the cell walls of plants. Whole, unprocessed grains, beans, fruits and vegetables all contain lots of fiber.

One Ayurvedic herb, psyllium seed, looks especially promising. Fiber is basically a food and aside from the occasional feeling of fullness, it rarely has any side effects.

Ancient Ayurvedic Diet Secrets to Lose Weight Naturally

Ayurvedic diet plans are an interesting way to eat healthy food and also lose weight. According to Ayurveda, everything is composed of five elements: air, water, fire, earth and space. These components combine to form the three doshas; vata, kapha and pitta, which account for the differences in the way out body responds to things.

Mindful eating and meditation after consumption helps to refine your taste buds thus destroy unhealthy cravings. Losing weight the Ayurvedic way is really one of the best one without any side effects since it is more of a lifestyle than a treatment. All the more Ayurveda promotes living by natural balanced diet. Ancient secrets are specifically made to keep your diet healthy and healing through eliminating wastes efficiently and promoting healthy digestion which naturally keeps you in an optimal shape and weight.

Get protein from soya, dals, grams etc. Non-vegetarian meals are not banned in Ayurveda, however, the present hormone pumped breed of poultry are certainly a "No". Small fish is permitted in its curry mode but not the fry. Processed sugar has no nutritional value but can excite your brain in a way that leads you to overeat. Eat meals which are easy to digest. This helps to improve metabolism and weight loss. Easily digested foods include steamed vegetables and soups.

Ayurveda offers a safe diet plan to get rid of weight and although there is absence of research in most areas it has a long trusted tradition of more than thousands of years.

Chapter 4: Six Tastes In Ayurvedic Diet

The ancient ayurvedic texts identify only six tastes. They are as follows:

1. Sweet flavor
2. Sour flavor
3. Salty flavor
4. Pungent flavor
5. Bitter flavor
6. Astringent flavor

Our tongue tip has it all! Proper nutrition majorly is dependent on the tastes we consume. To cure ailments, Ayurveda has been relying upon few lifestyle changes and on umpteen number of variations in food. Almost 80percentage of the ayurvedic medicines also comprise of some specific smells and tastes.

Sweet Flavor - The sweetness found in fruits, vegetables and other supplements of natural sugars help to build the tissues in our body. Additionally they are quite helpful in calming the nervous system.

It is from the amalgamation of water and the earth that the sweet taste emerges. These elements are quite soothing in nature. It is interesting to note that even milk and its foodstuffs along with the grains such as barley, wheat, and fruits such as bananas, mangoes etc are considered to be sweet.

The sweet taste increases body weight considerably. The dhatus or the vital tissues (bones, muscles etc,.) built only with the help of the sugar content in a diet. So you want a glowy skin, lustuorus hair and beautiful voice, start consuming foodstuffs which have sugar content in them!

[The sweet content aggravates 'kapha' body types, however is good for "vata" and "pitta" body types]

Sour Flavor – This is a flavor if its strong enough can possibly make you wink! The sour taste rinses the tissues from any impurities also in some amounts boosts the intake of minerals. This tangy taste is comprised of elements such as earth and fire.

The sour taste is found generally in yogurt, the fruits which are sour and in the foods which are fermented. It is helpful for digestion problems, making you heart stronger, relieving you of any acidity, and making your senses spiky!

[The sour taste is aggrevating for the pitta and kapha body types but is a balancing component for the vata body type.]

Salty Flavor – Salt is the essential nutrients which increases the taste in food prepared. Salt is comprises of the elements of water and fire. Like all other tastes, if used in excess, salt salt increases health risks.

Therefore, salt should be consumed in moderate proportions. It is interesting to note here that due to its inclination of attracting water, it helps in glowing skin.Consequently, salt intake in the body contributes to a healthy, development of a human body.

[This is beneficial for only the vata type bodies, but is the most aggravating for the pitta and kapha type bodies.]

Pungent Flavor – The elements of pungent tastes are a combination of air and water. This taste triggers the digestive system, relieves senses, increases the metabolism in a body also helps in fading away any muscle pain.

Ginger, garlic, onions black peppers all have this pungent tastes which helps in digestion and is also helps blood to flow without any difficulty.

[This is good for only the kapha constitution, as it aggravates the senses of vata and pitta body types]

Bitter Flavor – It has air and earth elements which is quite a combination for the human body. All greens (vegetables), herbs like the commonly found turmeric powder, coffee etc, comprise of this taste. These generally would be detoxifying with some antiseptic behavior.

[The vata type body needs to be essentially away from the bitterness, however, for kapha and pitta type bodies it would benefit them]

Astringent Flavor – The astringent taste comprises of the air and earth elements in it. With great soothing effects, can be a competitor of the sweet flavor. This flavor could be found in beans, pomegranates, dried fruits etc.

[Ideal for both pitta and kapha body types; is kind of an aggravating element for the vata body types.]

The ground rule is that a complete meal should comprise of all these elements for a body to have a healthy physique. Interestingly by following a diet balanced with all these flavors or tastes, over eating and carving for food could be also be avoided.

Chapter 5: Ayurveda Approach To Genital Herpes

Ayurveda approach to Genital Herpes Dosha theory which help in diagnosis of the diseases According to ayurveda three doshas or three energetic forces control the activities of the body. These doshas are 1. Vata 2. Pitta 3. Kapha VATA: The Vata dosha is the most important of the three doshas. It has been said in ayurveda classic books that " pitta , Kapha and all other body tissues are considered lame without assistance of VATA ." Vata dominates the lower part of the body, which is below umbilicus. The movements of body fluid, metabolism, elimination of waste products, semen ejaculation, pushing the fetus out of body, relaying stimulus to brain and response to organs and tissues, heart beat, respiration, body movements etc are assisted by VATA. Vata dominated regions are intestines, lumbar region, ears, bones and skin. Vata gets vitiated due to following reasons.

1. Controlling natural urges like urination, defecation, hunger, thirst, etc.

2. Late nights.

3. Irregular food habits.

4. Talking in a high pitch.

5. Over physical and mental exertion.

6. Consumption of spicy, dry, bitter foods.

7. Exposure to severe dry and cold climate. The opposites of above-mentioned reason normalize the vitiated vata. PITTA: The pitta dosha assists the body fire or Agni, which plays a major role in body's metabolic activities. The locations where pitta dominates are digestive system, skin, eyes, brain, and blood. Pitta maintains body temperature. The secretions like digestive juices pigments like melanin (bhrajaka pitta), hemoglobin (ranjaka pitta) are all types of pitta. Pitta is dominant in regions of Umbilicus, stomach, sweat,

lymph, blood, eyes and skin. Vata gets vitiated due to following reasons.

1. Excess consumption of spicy, sour, salty foods. 2. Consuming alcohol in excess.

3. Over exposure to hot sunny climate.

4. Short temperedness.

5. Using dried vegetables.

6. Indigestion of food. The opposites of above-mentioned reason normalize the vitiated pitta. KAPHA: Kapha provides bulk to body, lubrications, moistness, fertility, stability, strength, and memory. Helps in binding process wherever necessary. This is heaviest of all doshas. Kapha dominated regions are chest, neck, head, stomach, body fat, nose and tongue Kapha gets vitiated due to following reasons.

1. Sleeping in daytime.

2. Consuming sweets , chilled food, in excess.

3. Consuming fish, sesame, sugarcane, milk and milk products. The opposites of above-mentioned reason normalize the

vitiated kapha. When these doshas are in balanced condition the body remains healthy. If these doshas get imbalanced the body succumbs to diseases. Doshas get imbalanced frequently due to change in climate, seasons, lifestyles, diet etc. The treatment is to bring back the doshas to normalcy and expel the toxin or ama produced during the imbalanced condition. Causes of Genital Herpes Herpes is caused by a virus the herpes simplex virus (HSV), which belongs to the same family of viruses that cause chickenpox. There are two types of herpes simplex viruses

1. Herpes simplex type 1 (HSV-1) and mostly causes oral herpes

2. Herpes simplex type 2 (HSV-2). And mostly causes genital herpes However, both type-1 and type-2 can occur in the genitals, oral area or both. Due to unhealthy life styles and diet the delicate balance between doshas get disturbed. This disturbs the body fire or Agni. (Agni is

the body fire, which is responsible for transformation of one substance to another. It breaks down the food substances, eliminates toxins and wastes, maintains body temperature, and resists the invasion of microbes by maintaining strong body immunity. The body fire, which is assisted by balanced doshas, digests the food completely to form Pakwa Anna rasa (the liquid form of food which is completely digested by digestive enzymes), which is ready to get absorbed by body tissues. According to ayurveda Pakwa Anna Rasa nourishes the body and its components to keep the body devoid of diseases.

But when body fire is impaired there will be an incomplete digestion of food forming Apakwa Rasa (indigested food). The indigested food fails to nourish the body components leading to lowered body resistance.) The disturbed Agni fails to digest the food and toxins get accumulated in body due to improper metabolism. Accumulation of toxins reduces the body immunity and paves the way for invasion by microbes. When a person who has low immunity comes in contact with HSV virus, heshe gets the genital or oral herpes. Unhealthy lifestyle

1. Over eating

2. Sleeping in afternoons.

3. Over physical exertion.

4. Over mental exertion

5. Consuming food frequently even when not hungry.

6. Constant exposure to hot sunny climates

Unhealthy diet Excessive consumption of:

1. Salty, sour, hot, spicy food.
2. Sour curds
3. Alcohol.
4. Cheese
5. Charred and overcooked food.
6. Sesame, Bengal gram, horse gram, sesame oil, rice flour, garlic, fish.

Opposite foods

1. Curds, salt, mushrooms, bamboo shoots, sour fruits, meat, prawn, pork, should not be consumed with milk. The above-mentioned foods should not be consumed by mixing one item with another.

2. Sprouts, honey and milk should not be consumed with meat and fish.

3. Fish & milk: fish &sugarcane juice; jaggery & pork; honey & pork; milk & mango; banana & milk; are opposite foods.

The Transmission Of genital Herpes A person can get genital herpes in following conditions

1. If he is sexual active and when he performs sex (oral or genital) with infected partners.

2. A person who has oral herpes transmits herpes to genital organs of a partner during oral sex and a person who has genital herpes transmits this to his partner

during coitus when they have a genital contact.

3. The disease gets transmitted when mucous membrane comes in contact with infected area. The disease gets transmitted mostly during active phase. But it may spread even during asymptomatic (when person is free of symptoms for a particular duration) phase. The virus needs a fluid media for its transportation. The body fluids like saliva, semen, vaginal tract secretions etc. Mucous membranes in mouth, vagina, urethra or open wounds facilitate the virus invasion due to their moistness. In Genital herpes there is an imbalance of all three doshas (VATA, PITTA, KAPHA), which in turn vitiate lasika (lymph), blood (rakta), muscle (mamsa) and skin (twacha). The imbalanced doshas vitiate skin and the immunity of skin cells is lowered. The virus attacks these weak cells and starts exhibiting symptoms on affected area.

Local symptoms

1. Pricking sensation
2. Edema

3. Pain

4. Feeling of constriction

5. A sensation of ant creeping

6. Many small eruptions gathering in a small area.

7. These eruptions or blisters burst soon with exudates. 8. These blisters will have different colors according to involvement of doshas. (Blackish red or blue in vata, red, yellow, copper colored in pitta, shades of white in kapha). The weakened body immune system tries to resist the virus invasion but fails to achieve the goal. In this futile attempt the following systemic symptoms are exhibited.

Systemic symptoms

1. Fever
2. Weakness
3. Indigestion
4. Impaired bowels
5. Increased frequency of urination.
6. Body pain.
7. Increased thirst. Imbalanced vata causes the symptoms like pain, swelling and body ache

The imbalanced pitta and vitiated blood and skin cause

1. Blisters
2. Change the color of skin
3. Cause burning sensation, and fever. The imbalanced kapha and vitiated lymph cause itching, tingling sensation. After the first attack the virus moves from skin through the nerve paths to base of the nerve and becomes inactive. Now the herpes infected person will be devoid of all symptoms. But the imbalance of doshas

still persists. Reactivation of Virus to cause outbreaks At unpredictable times, the virus becomes active. It multiplies and resurfaces on skin by traveling through the nerve path and exhibits the symptoms locally. The severity of symptoms of out break depends on the strength of body immunity. The pelvis or shroni, nerves and skin are dominated by vata. When vata gets vitiated due to precipitating factors, it reactivates the virus dormant in base of nerve end and the virus travel through nerve paths to reach the skin surface.

Precipitating Factors

As we know the outbreaks have few precipitating factors like

1. Excessive exposure to sun.

2. Illness,

3. Poor diet,

4. Emotional stress

5. Physical stress,

6. Friction,

7. Steroids

8. Menstruation.

9. Emotional stress.

10. Genital trauma and intercourse.

11. Repeated infections such as a cold or pneumonia. These factors increase vata and increased vata activates the virus, which is dormant. Low Immunity The systemically imbalanced doshas interfere with the body metabolism by vitiating the body fire (agni). This leads to indigestion and malassimilation of nutrients, which in turn causes poor immunity.

Due to decreased immunity the body fails to offer resistance to outbreaks. Ayurveda Tips to avoid outbreaks

Avoid

1. Spicy, sour, fried and junk food, which aggravates vata.

2. Precipitating factors.

3. Sleeping in afternoon.

4. Meat products over fried or deep fried in oil or fat.

5. Charred and overcooked food.

6. Consuming opposite food like fish and milk etc

7. Physical exertion after a meal

8. Taking bath immediately after exercise or heavy outdoor work. Include honey, pomegranate, and fruits of Emblica officinalis, legumes, dates and raisins in your diet. Practice Yoga and Meditation to control emotional disturbances Ayurveda References 1. Sushruta Samhita 2. Charaka Samhita 3. Madhava nidana 4. Ashtanga Sangraha 5. Yoga Ratnakara

Chapter 6: Ayurveda Strategies To Treat Viral Infections And Fever

As per Ayurveda, generator of your body temperature is situated in your forehead. The disturbance to regulate the body temperature is known as Jwara, and it is correlated to the therapeutic concepts of fever. In numerous cases, the fever relates to the internal temperature of the gastrointestinal tract and external temperature. Fever can be a symptom of another disease, and the fever is often classified into eight different categories, such as Kapha, Pitta, Vata-Pitta, Vata, Pitta-Kapha, Vata-Kapha, Aghantuja and Vata-Pitta-Kapha. It can be the symptom of an infectious disease and classified as the Pitta character.

Fever Management Rules

If you are suffering from fever, you should eat light food in the initial stage. Fasting is good for the treatment of illness because it stimulates the stomach to draw the heat away from your periphery to the middle by increase your digestive fire. Warm water is good to drink with the Pitta character and it is good to maintain a healthy balance in your stomach. It will be good to include warm liquid in your diets, such as sago, barley, and vegetable soup. Anything with astringent taste is prohibited to take at the initial stage of your fever.

You can use antipyretic medicines during the initial stage of fever, such as cooling medication will reduce the temperature of your stomach. Using cooling herbs for the treatment of fever will be good. The cooling herbs will help you to treat your fever.

General Treatment for Fever

You can use Sudarsana curna to treat fever, and you can take almost 1 to 2 grams of this compound twice a day. A simple formula with Vasaka leaf and Shukti Bhasma (10 percent) are used with warm water almost two times in a day.

Treatment of Seasonal Fever for Monsoon (Vataja Jwara)

This fever is concerned with the intensified function or reduces the control of the nervous system. The symptoms of this fever include throbbing or excited pulse, fluctuating fever, shivering, dry throat and lips, dryness feeling, astringent taste in your mouth and body ache. This fever is common in the monsoon season during afternoon and morning time. Other causes of vataja fever are mental agony, depression, natural urges (defecation, flaus, and urination), excessive exercise and laxatives misuse, etc. This fever can be treated easily in monsoon, but in another season, this fever can difficult to treat.

Vataja fever can be treated with diet and antipyretic herbs. You can use 1 to 2 grams of Sudarshana churna twice a day to treat this fever. You can use different herbs, such as Piper longum (Pippali), Cyperus rotundus (Nagarmotha) and Boerhavia difusa (Punarnava).

Seasonal Fever for Autumn

You can treat a seasonal fever with the aggravated function of your vein system. The symptoms of this fever include a bitter taste in your mouth, burning sensation, high fever, sweating, nausea, dizziness, and diarrhea. It is caused by the extra exposure to heat, excessive exercise and extra consumption of salty and pungent food. You should avoid the consumption of alcoholic beverages. In the summer season, this fever is easy to treat. In other seasons, this fever can be difficult to treat. You can use chandanadi vas and Sudarshan churna twice a day. You can take 2 grams of honey almost twice in a day.

Seasonal Fever for Spring (Kapha)

The Jwara fever is concerned with the function of your artery system. The symptoms of this fever include lethargy, nausea, coldness, heaviness, sweet taste in your mouth, problems in the respiration and discoloration of eyes. This fever is common for spring and cures your fever by avoiding cold beverages and foods. You can treat this fever with some herbs, such as Sudarshana churna, Phyllanthus emblica (Amalaki fruit), Terminalia chebula (Haritaki fruit) and Plumbago zeylanica (Chitraka herb).

Chapter 7: Foods To Eat For Your Dosha

Depending on your dosha, know what foods are right for you. As you know your Ayurveda body type (vata, pitta, and kapha), you will find out what foods you should eat.

Vata benefits from warm, oily and heavy food. Such qualities are important, and are more relevant than the individual foods. Some of the best vata foods are:

Warm milk – Preferably, drink it with a pinch of cardamom and powdered ginger.

Butter or clarified butter (ghee) - You can add it to any food item.

Ginger (fresh) - It's considered the best pungent spice. You can also make ginger tea or add ginger to your meals.

Cream of wheat or rice - You can add ginger, cardamom and ghee to it.

Almonds - Use boiling water to rinse them then remove the skin. Slightly roast the almonds in ghee.

Root vegetables like sweet potatoes, red beets, and carrots - You can cook and spice them up.

Sweet fruit - Examples are red grapes, figs and dates - It's best to eat room temperature fruits. Soak dried fruits first before eating them.

Chicken broth

Kichari - You can pair it with root vegetables, fresh ginger and ghee.

Pitta benefits from dry, cold and heavy foods. Examples are:

Milk with a pinch of cardamom

Clarified butter - Also called ghee, clarified butter has special properties that help decrease pitta – even though ghee is oily.

Steamed broccoli

Sunflower seeds

Lassi (12 cup plain yogurt and ½ cup cumin-flavored water)

Leafy greens and salads

Cucumber

Cold cereal

Legumes and lentils

Kichari (with coriander, fresh cilantro, and cumin)

Kapha benefits from light, hot and dry food. Some of the best kapha foods are:

Warm rye, millet, or buckwheat

Hot water with lemon, honey, and fresh ginger - In general, kapha does best with less food and the ginger-honey-lemon infusion can substitute for food.

Astringent fruit like persimmon, apricot and pomegranate

Kichari - Make it spicy with chili, pepper and fresh ginger.

Leafy greens like beet greens, kale and dandelion

Soymilk

Sprouts

Artichoke, green beans and cauliflower

Legumes and lentils

Brussels sprouts (steamed)

Everyone has the three doshas in them, just one or two isare more dominant. However, there are certain foods that every body type can enjoy. These include:

Kichari

Mung dal

Basmati rice

Green beans and asparagus

Berries, apricots, apples

Clarified butter

Cilantro and peas

Goat's milk

Sunflower seeds

Lassi (12 cup plain yogurt and ½ cup water with a pinch of coriander, ginger, and cumin)

Kichari

You may notice that kichari is a mainstay among all the foods to eat for the vata, pitta and kapha types. Why? Kichari is an Ayurveda dish, which is mainly used during and after panchakarma (detox procedures) or illness. It is also used during healing fasts and it's a healing, perfectly balanced food for the three doshas.

It's best to use organic ingredients, and you can consume kichari – if you prefer it – on a two- to three-week monofast diet. Kichari can harmonize the mind and body and regulate your blood chemistry.

Ingredients:

1 to 2 tablespoons ghee (clarified butter) or any healthy cooking oil

½ cup basmati rice

1 cup mung beans (yellow split beans or green whole mung beans)

2 teaspoons coriander, ground

1 teaspoon turmeric, ground

1 teaspoon each of fenugreek seeds, mustard seeds, and cumin seeds

1 to 3 teaspoons fresh ginger, grated

18 teaspoon of asafetida or hing (optional)

6 to 8 cups water

Organic vegetables (your choice). You can use any vegetables except onions, garlic, tomatoes, bell peppers, potatoes, and eggplant.

Rinse the rice and mung beans three times before cooking. Soak the beans one to eight hours. The process can help in eliminating gas formation.

In a deep pot over low to medium heat, melt the ghee or your choice of quality cooking oil. Add the grated ginger, mustard seeds, fenugreek and cumin. Sauté until slightly browned and not burnt.

Add the drained mung beans and rice and sauté for about 30 seconds more. Lower the heat. Add the hing, coriander and turmeric powders and sauté for 30 more seconds.

Add the water. The kitchari must be of soup consistency, so add more water as your see fit. Add the organic root vegetables. Cover the pot and simmer for 20 to 30 minutes. Add leafy greens. Cook further for 20 minutes more.

Serve. If you desire, add a little salt on top or Bragg's seasoning.

The world is your table. As long as you know the basic foods to eat for your dosha type and are familiar with the six tastes, you will know other kinds of food that belong to a certain taste even if they are not listed above. While the Ayurveda diet only requires you to follow a few simple rules, it is still important to learn more about the six tastes. Once you are already familiar with them, losing weight or attaining optimal health will be relatively easy.

Chapter 8: Ayurveda Secrets For Pure Energy And Contentment

In today's world of pollution, traffic and the unhygienic conditions surrounding us, people tend to get tired at a very fast pace. Upon feeling tired we automatically think of a strong and powerful energy drink thinking that this will be the one to boost back our energy level and let us carry out our tasks. For example, some dark chocolate or a food which has high nutritional value. The energy this food provides is however at that time effective but they are temporary and after a while we get back to again how we were before. For a permanent effect, there needs to be something that lasts for a much longer time. Therefore, as a healthy solution we provide you a few ayurvedic secrets for a much longer and better energy pertaining situation. Some of them are:

5. Having more than two meals a day without any snack in between: to stop eating snack and junk food is the best possible way to be healthy. Apart from that, it is advisable to have a hearty lunch, as day time digests our food in the best possible way. Having a snack or dinner at very late hours of the night makes it very difficult to lose weight; therefore this is not advisable as well.

6. Keep hydrated: it is commended to drink at least 10 litres or more water in a day. Water is a great drink for health. People who keep hydrated usually find its benefits to be extremely rewarding. It is advisable to drink hot water or normal water all throughout the day.

7. Eat those foods which possess energy: such as vegetables, namely the root ones which are mostly preferred like beetroots, carrots, potatoes etc. Other vegetables which have fiber in them are also recommended for example spinach. The oils which don't have unnecessary fats in them are highly recommended for instance olive oil, fish oil and ghee. And ayurvedic spread which consists of majority of vitamin E, vitamin B and many minerals.

8.Intake of a balanced meal: one of the most important thing to keep in mind when trying to stay healthy is that you have to think about the food you are eating and the time intervals between each meal. Having a balanced meal, which is divided according to the ingredients each meal, possesses and the timing between them is truly a good sign of being healthy. An example of a balance meal on a plate is meat ¼, salad ¼, dressing ¼, and steamed vegetables ¼. You can see that each of the ingredients mentioned is precise, and this has to be followed three times a day. Eating junk at odd times and eating meals even with improper timing and rest to the stomach is bound to create trouble for your health.

9. Speed up digestion: for some people the digestion of the meal is not very hard enough. But for some people digesting food is a bit different and may take up longer. An ayurvedic secret of speeding up the digestion process includes some natural steps to follow. Having 2 glasses of water before starting your meal helps in speeding up the digestion process and hydrates the stomach before the actual process of digestion. A nap or rest is recommended after lunch time specifically which aids in the digestion process. Cardamom, ginger, cumin and coriander if taken with the meal or even before the meal provide considerable amount of energy to the cells which eventually boost up the digestion process. All these spices and products are easily available, infact they are so common that they can be readily found in everyone's home. So you don't even need to worry about going out and buying.

10. Exercising: ayurvedic principles involve many benefits for those who perform exercise. Exercising should be a vital part of one's life accompanied by some fresh air. Taking a morning stroll in the park and breathing deeply through the nose makes the air go inside the body and gives energy to the body. Exercising is extremely beneficial and has some amazing benefits for a person, exercising reduces the risk of some deadly disease and illness, it prevents diabetes from occurring, lowers the risk of deaths, and even prevents cancer, which is a deadly disease associated with rapid growth of cells.

Chapter 9: Benefits Of Ayurveda Diet As Per Your Body Constitution

Nobody would like to get sick as this would mean having to be absent for work or not being able to do the activities that you love. Unfortunately, very few people know anything or much about Ayurveda and how Ayurveda diet keeps people healthy.

Ayurveda is an ancient 5000 year old wisdom that treats each individual as a unique body and offers unique diet, herbs, and other remedies for that particular individual. It provides a manual living for a healthy life and is intended for preventing illnesses like heart disease, hypertension and arthritis. Ayurveda considers an overweight or an underweight person as one who is more prone on catching diseases. To prevent such a thing, it recommends a unique Ayurveda diet suitable to the individual's psycho-physiological body type. The unique diet will help bring the body to a healthy state with an optimum weight.

If you are looking forward to using Ayurveda in your everyday life, try following an Ayurveda diet for clean eating recommended as per your psycho-physiological body type. An Ayurvedic practitioner can help you with creating an Ayurveda diet. Eating more than your body needs before the next meal can produce toxins along with fat deposits. Also, by eating foods outside of your diet list of foods can create imbalance and toxins in the body.

Have a balanced diet and a regular meal time. Uncontrolled eating habits contribute to gaining weight, which you must avoid. Also, learn how to make combinations of food items the proper way. Eating incompatible food items at the same meal slows down the digestive process of your body, making you grow fatter.

Along with other Ayurveda health tips, following your Ayurveda diet each day is the most important health tip. Some of the very basic health Ayurveda tips that apply to everyone are:

- Always start each day with a glass of warm water
- Avoid eating raw vegetables and raw foods and of course avoid over cooking as well
- Use ginger or cumin in recipes to aid digestion
- Do not drink iced or cold water before, during or right after the meal
- Perform 1-2 times per week oil massage using sesame oil
- Make a daily routine and follow it religiously
- Introduce meditation and yoga exercises in your routine, if you are not doing already

One additional adjustment suggested by Ayurveda is to adjust the Ayurveda diet based on seasons. This involves fine tuning the diet which is already based on the body's psycho-physiological constitution. Every one's body constitution has its corresponding seasonal herbs, foods, and oils that will enhance the body metabolism and ensure proper digestion. Once you have your diet plan all set, you can use it for life to maintain good health.

Thank you for your time & attention to this subject. Please read more and share with your friends the Simple Secrets to Good Health with Clean Eating.

Chapter 10: Hair Fall

Hair fall sucks. We've all had to deal with it at some point. And with chunks of hair falling out, it is hard not to stress out, which causes more hair loss. It's a vicious cycle and one that seems never ending. But you'll be happy to know that there is light at the end of the tunnel and ayurvedic remedies can help you get to that light sooner.

Ayurvedic treatments are a popular choice among many women for hair loss because they incorporate natural ingredients and have been an effective cure for hair fall since ancient times. Following is a list of 12 ayurvedic remedies for hair loss and hair regrowth, but before we get into that let's look at how Ayurveda can help tackle hair fall.Ayurvedic research on hair growth is extensive and well structured which makes it easy for practitioners to pinpoint the cause of hair fall and treat it accordingly.

According to Ayurveda, hair type is directly related to body type and is systematically classified into three categories; Vata, Pitta, and Kapha. Each hair type has distinct features, and hence there are multiple reasons for hair loss which vary from person to person.

Hair loss is caused because of pitta dosha. Pitta governs our metabolism and digestion. A balanced Pitta leads to a healthy body and mind. It controls our general well being. Once you identify the reasons of pitta dosha, it becomes easier to correct it. Typically, bad eating habits, anxiety, and stress cause pitta dosha, which in turn leads to hair loss. Excessive consumption of tea, coffee, alcohol, meat, fried and spicy food can cause an imbalance in pitta.

Apart from Pitta Dosha, other reasons for hair loss according to Ayurveda are hormonal imbalances in men and women, stress, lack of sleep, improper diet, intoxicating substances, dandruff or fungal infections and diseases like lupus or diabetes amongst others. Ayurvedic hair regrowth solutions address these core issues promoting hair regrowth.Ayurveda addresses 3 key concepts of care during the treatment, namely; Nidana (diagnostic measures), Ahar (food that can be used as preventive medicine) and Chikitsa (support and self-care).

1. Bhringraj—The King Of Herbs

Translated, Bhringraj means "king of herbs." True to its name, not only does it help promote hair growth, but it also reverses balding. It can be used to prevent premature graying. The herb is commonly available in powdered form and as an oil. It has a calming effect when applied to the scalp and helps insomniacs sleep better.

You Will Need:

A handful of Bhringraj Leaves

OR

5-6 tbsp Dried Bhringraj Powder

Processing Time

20 minutes

Method

Blend the leaves with some water to get a consistent paste. If you cannot find Bhringraj leaves, mix 5-6 tablespoons of dried bhringraj powder with some water to get a thick consistent paste.

Apply the paste to your scalp and hair and leave it in for 20 minutes.

Wash off with shampoo.

How Often?

Thrice a week.

You can also use this in combination with other ayurvedic ingredients such as amla and tulsi. Alternatively, you can give yourself a scalp massage with bhringraj oil thrice a week to promote hair growth.

2. Amla—The Indian Gooseberry

Amla is not only used as an ayurvedic solution for hair fall, but also an effective treatment for purifying blood and treating indigestion. This conditioning ingredient improves scalp health by tackling dandruff and scalp aggravation. When used in combination with shikakai, it acts as a natural dye that imparts a natural brown color.

You Will Need

5-6 tbsp Amla Powder

5-6 tbsp Water

Processing Time

30 minutes

Process

In a bowl, combine the ingredients to get a thick, smooth paste.

Section your hair and start applying this paste to your scalp and hair.

Leave it in for 30 minutes and then wash off with shampoo.

How Often?

Thrice a week.

You can also add shikakai powder to this mix by soaking amla and shikakai powder in warm water overnight. Alternatively, you can also extract amla juice from the fruit and use the liquid for scalp and hair treatment.

3. Neem:

For years, neem has been used to treat skin conditions and hair loss. Regular use of neem on the scalp improves blood circulation and strengthens the roots which, in turn, promotes hair growth. Neem is also used to treat dandruff and lice. When the scalp is affected by dryness, scaliness, dandruff, eczema, psoriasis and excessive sebum—the hair roots get damaged. This causes hair loss. Neem helps battle these conditions, soothes the scalp and promotes healthy hair growth.

You Will Need

A handful of Neem Leaves

2 cups Water

Processing Time

5 minutes

Process

Boil the neem leaves in water for 15 minutes and then set it aside to cool.

Once the solution is cool, strain the liquid.

Collect the neem infused water in a jug and set it aside.

Wash and condition your hair and pour the neem infused water through it as a final rinse

Do not rinse your hair any further.

How Often?

Thrice a week.

Alternatively, you can make a paste of dried neem powder and water, and leave it in your hair for 30 minutes before shampooing.

4. Ritha (Soap Nuts)

Ritha or soap nuts have been used by women for centuries as a natural shampoo. When used regularly, ritha promotes hair growth, improves texture and volume. Because of how mild it is, the natural ingredient can be used to cleanse your hair every day without it stripping away the natural oils from your scalp.

You Will Need

A handful of Soap Nuts

2 cups Water

Processing time

10 minutes

Process

Soak the soap nuts overnight in 2 cups of warm water.

In the morning, boil the soap nuts in the same water for about 15 minutes and then set it aside to cool.

Strain the cooled solution and collect the liquid in a jug.

Rinse your hair with water and then pour half of the soap nut solution through your hair.

Massage your hair for 5 minutes and then rinse with water.

Repeat with the remaining soap nut shampoo. The solution will start to form a slight lather at this point.

How Often?

On alternate days.

Chapter 11: What Is Insomnia?

One in four people around the globe suffer from lack of sleep insomnia and Ayurveda has a solution to the problem. There're tried and tested methods that have worked wonder to many people around the world. According to Ayurveda insomnia is a problem with low Kapha Dosha and high Vata Dosha. All factors leading to these two dosha stages can cause or worsen insomnia. First let us look at the reasons that cause lack of sleep in a person and how it can be remedied.

Causes for insomnia

When sleep eludes a person, even the smallest noise like ticking of the clock or water dropping from the tap literally pounds into the head. Tossing and turning becomes a common phenomenon during night bringing lethargy during daytime. This leads to several health problems like acidity, high blood pressure, headache, depression and aggression.

Some of the common reasons for the manifestation of this problem are:

• Effects of medications:

If a person is kept on medication, then the sleep pattern sometimes get disturbed.

• Erratic Lifestyle :

The body has an in-built body clock which works according to the biorhythm of the body. Irregular sleeping habits disrupts the natural sleeping cycle of the body causing biological imbalance in the body. Too much partying and keeping awake late into the night confuses the body clock and gives the wrong signal to the brain resulting in insomnia.

• Nature of work:

When your work compels you to keep awake during the night compulsorily, your body clock reverses and you automatically start sleeping during the day hours while you keep awake during the night. This generally happens when you're working in a factory or hospital wherein you are doing the night shift. Many IT professionals who work at night have had trouble with their health leading to impotency and erectile dysfunction as well.

• Stress:

Not the least, it is stress that keeps a person awake during night. As you lie awake in your bed, thinking about the mistakes you did during the day or the prospects missed, your subconscious mind starts preparing for counter actions to be taken for those past decisions. It starts strategizing on the plan of action which activates the nervous system and pushes the sleep away.

• Eating habits:

Eating food which causes the sugar to increase in the body also causes insomnia. Keep the food pyramid in mind while eating. Eating a heavy breakfast and a light dinner before going to bed helps a lot in fighting this problem. Even if you're on healthy weight loss diets, see to it that you eat wholesome food that induces sleep.

How to overcome insomnia

Besides Ayurveda there are several other holistic methods to overcome insomnia. Listening to soulful music, chants, hymns, yoga, meditation and hypnosis are some of the methods that can give you a good night's sleep.

Yoga – Yoga is the panacea of all ills. The poses asanas are very effective in curing sleep issues as well as other illnesses. Forward bend uttanasana, corpse poseShavasana, cow pose bitilasana, Marjariasana are some of the poses that stretch your back and neck to relax your body and let the blood flow freely to the head. This automatically induces sleep.

Exercise – Running, jogging, skipping and working out at the gym can help in blood circulation throughout the body and this can tire you inducing sleep. Even a quiet walk at night after dinner can aid in digestion and encourage good sleep.

Control your diet – Instead of gorging on fried and sugary foods go in for a bowl of fresh soup with veggies for dinner. Even green smoothies will do. Not only are they rich in iron they are rich in fiber that helps in digestion too.

Listening to soulful music helps the mind to relax and sleep peacefully. The lilting sound of musical instruments and the soulful voice of the singer act like aphrodisiac and lull you to sleep.

Meditation stills the mind and offers peace and tranquility which in turn helps to have a good night's rest.

Hypnosis is another best method to overcome sleep disorder. You can also resort to self hypnosis. This penetrates deep into your subconscious and gives positive affirmations and suggestions. The amazing aspect of this theory is that not only you eradicate the problem out of your system; you are also able to go to the root cause of it manifesting in your body, in the first place. This happens because hypnosis works deep into the innermost recesses of the mind.

Affirmations

A single line affirmation like this can work wonders, "With each breath I take, I feel more and more relaxed". And then continue to affirm and relax each and every body part by affirming, "With each breath I take, my eyes are more relaxed, my forehead is more relaxed", and so on and so forth and find yourself going to sleep effortlessly without having to count the boring sheep!

Besides all the above mentioned methods, Ayurveda has cure for insomnia that can help you to sleep well without any disturbance. Read on to know about it.

Chapter 12: Demon-Riddance

Every imbalance, every disease, was assumed to be caused by sin (Anglo-Saxon word meaning "error"), and

engineered by demons affecting the mind, and causing one's own mind to turn against one's own body.

Prem Rawat said that when you take away the blocks, everything flows.

I will translate this into ayurveda by saying, take away the sins (repent) and remove the interference (remove the demons affecting the mind) – remove the interference that interferes with automatic unconscious regeneration and maintenance, then all four lower bodies are regenerated and maintained.

This is what the Vedic healers believed also.

Many types of demons were identified. Remember, these gained admittance into the body (or are sent to the sinner as punishment) through aberrations in the mind, or aberrations in the pattern of spiritual cognition.

During good health, these mental or spiritual patterns are regulated by following moral principles, and by ayurvedic practices.

Sometimes the patient's healthy mental pattern might have been disrupted by seiðr, or psychic attack by a sorcerer. This would also be karmic; or else the victim became vulnerable to the sorcerer by making some mistake or sin.

Or, if they didn't make a mistake, the victim was deficient in performing actions that would strengthen them spiritually. They didn't do enough of something, to make them strong and protected.

This spiritual strength, if they had gotten it, would have protected them against the attempted seiðr. In other words, the person being attacked wasn't strong enough, and was not relying on a strong enough divine protector, or else they neglected to form a strong enough tie to that divine protector.

Thus they became vulnerable to seiđr, and thus demons were able to enter in and block the automatic flowing of the victim's healing energy.

One type of demon, mentioned in the Vedas, is a demon associated with general internal disease that was to be found in Mankind and in cattle.

Themodus operandi, of this particular type of demon, was to enter and possess every part of the body, to disintegrate the limbs, to cause fever in the limbs, heartache, and pains in all parts of the body.

Many types of demon speak like a child and like an adult:

- The unknown yáksma
- The royal yáksma – rájayáksma

Often these are associated with other entities that cause internal disease. Many of these other entities require separate mantras for their removal:

• The jaundice group. These are treated as a single phenomenon in a mantra found in Atharva Veda 19.44.2

☐ Jāyānya

☐ Jaundice

☐ Disintegration of limbs

☐ Visálpaka

• Takmán, a cause of fever – mantras found in Atharva Veda 5.4.9, 5.30.16

• Demons causing diseases of the head – mantra found in Atharva Veda 9.8.1

• Balása -- mantra found in Atharva Veda 9.8.10

• Visalpá, vidradhá, vātīkārá, and alají, -- mantra found in Atharva Veda 9.8.20 (c.f.9.8.5)

• Kṣetriyá, a hereditary disease, or hereditary disease -- mantra found in Atharva Veda 2.10.5 and 6 [Note I use here the "ş" with the cedilla in lieu of one with a dot beneath it, because there was not one available in my word processor. I do not know whether or not the pronunciation would be the same.]

There is a celestial personage known by the name Yama. Yama is also known outside of Indian lore as "the angel of death. It has been suggested that Yama is the same as the "I Am" who spoke to Moses. In the olden days, "I Am" would have been pronounced as "Ee-Ahm.

As the angel of death, Yama has often been found to associate with demons:

•Nírṛti, who is a demonesstroll of destruction – mantra found in Atharva Veda 8.1.21

•Grāhi, a demon of seizure – mantra found in Rig Veda 10.161.1, in Atharva Veda 3.11.1 and 20.96.6

Another set of demons originates in the relatives of the bride, and follows the wedding-procession. These are found in

Rig Veda 10.85.31, which is the same as Atharva Veda 14.2.10.

Some demons are sent by God, or by the servants of God, because of énas, which means a mistake, such as a dishonest man pressing the juice of soma, or allowing a cow's hair to become hurt.

For each type of demon, there is a plant or plants to be held in the hand of the bhiṣái, and stroked or waved over the patient, while mantras were recited, quite likely with the bhiṣái attending to his own breath.

This combination of actions caused the demons to leave the patient's body, and to fly away with the birds.

A lead amulet dispels the demon downward, an ointment removes it from the patient's limbs. A varaṇa-tree amulet restrains the Devas from dispatching demons toward the patient.

Since the demon was sent by God, or by God's servants, the Devas, they have the power to destroy it. The most helpful Devas, to this end, are Agni, Savitṛ, Vāyu, and Aditya. Water is also used. Smoke of the gulgulú-plant disperses certain demons.

Chapter 14: The Characteristics Of Kapha

Dooshas Are –

- Snigdhna – slick, unctuous
- Sheeta – cool
- Guru – overwhelming
- Manda – gentle, thick
- Shlakshna – smooth, clear
- Mrutsna – vile, jam
- Sthira – strength, stability

Oiliness is the characteristics of Kapha.

What is the Ayurvedic perspective of structure and elements of body?

Universe and additionally human body are comprised of five essential components all in all called 'Pancha Mahabhuta'.

These are Aakash (Ether), Vayu (Air), Agni (Fire), Aapa (Water) and Prithvi (Earth). The 6th obligatory segment of life is Atma (life soul) without which life stops.

The human body is comprised of Dooshas (Bio-humors), Dhatus(Body lattice) and Malas (excretable items)

Vata, Pitta and Kapha, known as Tridoshs are physiological elements of the body which are in charge of doing every one of the elements of the body.

Dhatus

Ayurveda clarifies around 7 body tissue segments which shape the physical body. The working of body tissue is controlled by Tri Dooshas.

These seven body tissues are called as "Dhatus" in Ayurveda.

These are

1.Rasa (Plasma)

2. Rakta (Blood cells)

3. Mamsa (Muscular tissue)

4. Meda (Fatty tissue)

5. Asthi (Bony tissue)

6. Majja (Bone marrow)

7. Shukra (Hormonal and different emissions of genital).

Rasa Dhatu – The Rasa is created not long after assimilation. It is the pith some portion of the food that circles everywhere throughout the body and supports all the body tissues. It is horribly contrasted with plasma some portion of blood. It's essential capacity is Preenana – to support all the body tissues.

It is controlled by Kapha Dooshas. Generally Kapha Dooshas increment causes increment of Rasa Dhatu. Furthermore, Kapha diminish prompts Rasa Dhatu diminish.

Rakta Dhatu – It is contrasted straightforwardly and blood and its part. It is framed by getting the support from Rasa

Dhatu. Its fundamental capacity is Jeevana – exciting. It is straightforwardly related with Pitta Dooshas. Pitta Dooshas increment prompts Rakta increment and the other way around.

Mamsa Dhatu – It is contrasted and muscle tissue. It gets its food from Rakta Dhatu. Its fundamental capacity is Lepana – It offers shape to the body parts and it adheres to the bones, helping in locomotor exercises. It is controlled by Kapha Dooshas. Typically Kapha Dooshas increment and decline prompts Mamsa Dhatu increment and diminishing separately.

Meda Dhatu – It is contrasted with fat tissue. It gets sustained by Mamsa Dhatu. Its fundamental capacity is Snehana – oil. Its expansion and lessening is impacted by Kapha Dooshas. Thus, Kapha Dooshas prevailing individual is typically rich in fat tissue.

Asthi Dhatu – It is contrasted with bone tissue. It gets fed by Meda Dhatu. Its fundamental capacity is Dharana – to hold the body up straight. It is affected by Vata Dooshas. Be that as it may, Vata Dooshas increment prompts Asthi Dhatu diminish and Vata Dooshas diminish prompts Asthi Dhatu increment. This is the reason, in maturity, when Vata is expanded, bone tissue degeneration happens.

Majja Dhatu – It is contrasted with bone marrow and all the tissue that fill bone depression. For instance, eye tissue is additionally considered as Majja. Some likewise consider mind tissue additionally as framed by Majja Dhatu. Its fundamental capacity is Poorana – to fill in the bone holes. Its expansion and diminishing is controlled by Kapha Dooshas.

Shukra Dhatu – It is contrasted and male and female conceptive framework and its discharges. Its primary capacity is Garbhotpadana – multiplication. It is controlled by Kapha Dooshas. It gets support from Majja Dhatu.

Agni (Metabolic fire) is in thirteen unique structures and does the entire digestion of the body.

The waste results of the body which are excretable are delivered in the body as bye-results of digestion. These are known as malas which incorporate pureesh (excrement), Sweda (sweat) and Mutra (pee).

All biotransformations inside the body happen through Srotases (body channels) which are the locales for activity of Agni.

What is the fundamental theory of wellbeing, sickness and treatment in Ayurveda?

According to Ayurveda, "Wellbeing" is a condition of harmony of ordinary elements of Dooshas, Dhatus, malas and Agni with charmed body, brain and soul. It implies that when Dosh-Dhatu-Malas and Agni are continually in a condition of utilitarian harmony, then the wellbeing is kept up. Generally twisting of the harmony comes about into infections. Whimsical way of life is accepted to be one of the essential causes behind the disappointment of instrument of looking after balance.

How is analysis done in Ayurveda?

There are three principle techniques said in Ayurveda for diagnosing the Dooshas unevenness and ailment handle in a man. They are –

Darsana Pareeksha - By watching the patient's physical signs and manifestations, case – shade of skin, hair, eyes, conduct, body condition and so on.

Prasna Pareeksha - By soliciting minute inquiries in regards to the unevenness from each Dooshas

Sparsana Pareeksha – By heartbeat analysis, palpation, percussion and auscultation are incorporated into this technique

Indicative systems in Ayurveda are two dimensional; one is expected to set up the state and sort of pathology and second to choose the method of treatment to be connected. The previous infers examination of the patient and make distinctive examinations to analyze the illness substance. Assessment, palpation, percussion and cross examination are the primary methods of physical examination. The second kind of examination is to survey the quality and physical status of the individual so that as needs be the sort of administration required could be arranged. For this examination of Prakriti (Body constitution), Saar (Tissue quality), Samhnan (build), Satva (Mental quality), Satamya (particular versatility), Aaharshakti (consume less calories consumption limit), Vyayaam shakti (practice limit) and Vaya (age) is finished. On the premise of this examination the individual is chosen to have Pravar BAL (astounding quality), Madhyam Bal (direct quality) or Heen Bal (low quality).

Chapter 15: Increasing Breast Milk Production:

• Breast milk is a very important nutritional source for babies as it:

o Strengthens the immune system

o Increases memory and IQ

• Low milk supply can put the baby at risk of malnutrition

Causes:

• The milk production can be limited due to:

o Any illness

o Consuming birth-control pills

• Certain hormonal disorders

• Infrequent breastfeeding by the mother due to cracked or painful nipples

Natural home remedy using fenugreek seeds and cowgoatcamel milk:

1. Take some washed fenugreek seeds

2. Crush them to powder

3. Mix 1 tbsp of this powder in milk from a cow, goat or camel

4. Drink 3 glasses of this milk every day

- It stimulates the milk producing glands. Diabetic and asthmatic women should avoid this remedy.

Natural home remedy using drumstick juice:

1. Drink ½ glass of drumstick juice every day

- This will stimulate the mammary glands. It will also open up veins around the breast, which will

increase the supply of milk.

Tips:

- Keep the body hydrated by drinking water and juices through the day

- Have a nutritious diet and increase your daily calorie intake

- Using a warm compress on your breast before the feeding session increases the blood supply in the

region

Fibroids:

- Fibroids is a condition which affects women
- Tumors develop within and outside the uterus
- The condition is usually detected only after the tumours have grown in size
- Tumors shrink after menopause, due to decline in the level of reproductive hormones

Symptoms to look for:

- Abdominal discomfort
- Backache
- Frequent urination
- Pain during:

o Menstruation cycle

o Bowel movements

o Sexual intercourse

Causes:

- Obesity
- Alteration in genes
- Increase in level of hormones like estrogen and progesterone

Natural home remedy using milk, turmeric, coriander powder and triphala:

1. Turmeric soothes any inflammation while coriander purifies the blood.

Triphala, an ayurvedic herb, rejuvenates the body.

2. Take 1 glass warm milk
3. Add 1 tsp turmeric powder
4. Add 1 tsp coriander powder
5. Add 1 tsp triphala powder
6. Mix well
7. Drink 2 times a day

Tips:

- Include kidney beans and black-eyed beans in your daily diet as they help reduce the estrogen levels

• Fish like salmon and tuna have anti-inflammatory properties and help counter fibroids

Yeast Infection (Thrush):

• Yeast infection is commonly known as thrush

• It can affect any part of the body, but it primarily affects:

o Under arms

o Area between toes

o Genital area

• This condition affects both men and women

• Women usually develop this infection in their vagina

Symptoms to look for:

• Itching

• Discomfort during intercourse

• Burning sensation during urination

Causes:

- Yeast are microorganisms which are present in our body. An increase in the level of yeast leads to this infection. The level of acid, which keeps yeast in check, dips during:

o Pregnancy

o Menstruation

o Diabetes

o Intake of birth control pills

Natural home remedy using aloe vera:

1. Aloe vera gel is very effective
2. Take an aloe vera leaf
3. Peel off the skin
4. Extract the gel from inside
5. Apply this gel on the infected area
6. Leave it for 30 min
7. Wash it off with water
8. Do this twice a day

Natural home remedy using coconutcinnamon oil:

1. Apply coconut or cinnamon oil 2-3 times a day

2. Both oils have anti-fungal properties

Natural home remedy using yogurt:

1. Soak cotton in yogurt

2. Apply it on the infected area

3. Leave it for 30 min

4. Do this twice a day

Tips:

• For non-vaginal infections, apply garlic paste directly on the infected parts

• Do not scratch the infected area

Female Sterility (Infertility):

• Female sterility or infertility refers to a condition in which a woman is unable to conceive

• Ability to conceive reduces with age. Women find it difficult to get pregnant after 35 years of age

Symptoms to look for:

• Irregular menstrual cycle

Causes:
- Ageing
- Being overweight or underweight
- Excessive smoking
- Alcohol consumption
- Illicit drugs
- Endometriosis
- Any blockage in the fallopian tubes

Natural home remedy using banyan tree bark and milk:

1. Take a small piece of banyan tree bark, available in ayurvedic stores
2. Wash thoroughly
3. Remove the outer-covering
4. Leave the bark in the sun for 1 hr
5. Crush it to a powder
6. Take 2 tbsp of this powder
7. Add to 1 glass of lukewarm milk
8. Mix well
9. Drink on an empty stomach
10. Do this for 6 months

Do not try this remedy during periods.

Natural home remedy using shatavari powder and milk:

1. Take 1 tbsp of shatavari powder, an ayurvedic herb
2. Add to 1 glass of milk
3. Mix well
4. Drink every day at bedtime

Natural home remedy using ashwagandha powder:

1. Take 1 glass of warm water
2. Add 1 tbsp of ashwagandha powder, an ayurvedic herb
3. Mix well
4. Drink 2 times a day
5. Add honey for taste

Tips:

- Consult your doctor before eating seafood. Fish contain mercury which can lead to birth defects
- Avoid consuming caffeine. It is present in tea and coffee

- Avoid consuming fast food, drinking alcohol and smoking

Chapter 15: Root Cause Of Sickness

What is disease? Why do we get sick? Why does imbalance occur? Are body constitutions just a stroke of luck we receive at birth? These questions are what Ayurveda tried to answer and understand through years of study. Ayurveda principles understand that when there is balance, there is also absence of disease and vice versa, when there is imbalance, disease is present. Learning the principles of Ayurveda, to a wise man means that he is aware that learning to balance his doshas and establishing this balance means a healthy constitution.

Understanding Diseases

The ancient knowledge of Ayurveda and according to the old age spiritual tradition of India, there are two causes of diseases.

The first root of disease is believed to be from biological or physical causes. This means that there is simply an imbalance of the biological humors which are the main sources of physical health. Therefore, treatment can be in the form of diet alteration, herbs, yogic postures and body work. Though, in some extreme cases, surgery and drug medicines are really needed as intervention in order to regain balance.

The second root cause of disease is believed to be from karmic causes. Karma simply means is the effects of the wrong actions one has done in his life. Karmic causes may also be from spiritual or psychological causes. To further elaborate, karmic cause can also be from problems in relationships, wrong occupation, emotional difficulties and spiritual reasons. The treatment for these diseases is mostly a change in perspective, attitude in life, reactions and life-style. Thus root of disease also stems from a person who is not living his purpose in life or not being wary of his spiritual will in life. This is what is known in Sanskrit as one's „dharma.' It is believed that diseases can also arise from one's wrong actions from his previous life, especially those that have caused misfortune or abuse to other beings. This can be from misuse of power or resources.

These karmic causes of diseases usually require some form of sacrifice or atonement (an inner process or rectification). Usually, Ayurveda suggests the practice of Yoga and spiritual therapy in the form of gem use, prayers, mantras, rituals and meditations in order for healing to take place. Though these remedies may appear „medieval' to some, they are believed to reflect a deeper level of understanding one's mind and body and to the definition of healing as well. This is because these types of healing takes into consideration the subtler aspects of one's being, meaning to say, it is holistic and goes beyond the physical.

In Ayurveda, it is believed that the human being is made up of three bodies namely:

the physical, the astral and the causal. In Western terms, it is called the body, mind and soul. The way of treatment in Western medicine also tends to focus on the physical (body) because it uses the system of diagnosis and treatment but also considers the other two. While in Ayurveda, many of its methods take into consideration the energy field beyond the physical body and also the level of consciousness behind it. This is because Ayurveda believes that most diseases involve an imbalance both in the spiritual and physical factors and of course, will require treatment in both areas as well.

The importance of one's knowledge of the doshashumors and constitutions plays an important role when it comes to understanding the root of diseases. Disease proneness or tendencies has a lot to do with the constitutions. **For example,** Vatas are prone to constipation more than Pittas and Kaphas.

Pittas, on the other hand are most likely to have gall bladder and liver disorders than the ones from the other two constitutions.

Kaphas, will most likely have tonsillitis, sinusitis bronchitis as their diseases more than any other type of disease.

Secret Of Health

1. Balancing the tastes

Food plays a great role in the overall health of a person. Food preference help the doshas to be kept in balance, thus is considered a secret in health. As the old saying goes, 'too much of anything is simply bad, 'same applies to the food that one eats. One should keep in mind that too much intake of sweets damages the spleen or pancreas. Whereas, too much sour damages the liver while too much bitter may give heart problems. Preference for pungent taste dries up the lungs while salty food destroys the liver. Inside the body, sweets build up toxins, bitter cause cold which is a perfect environment for a number of diseases, salty cause looseness and pungent is the root of burning. One aiming for a good health should always keep this is mind.

2. Getting to know Agni

Agni can be defined as the biological fire or heat energy that is responsible for metabolism. Metabolism, on the other hand, plays a very important role in the overall health of a person. It is the collection of every chemical reaction that takes place in every cell in the human body. Therefore, metabolism is the one that converts the food that one eats to fuel or energy that is needed by the cells organsbodily systems to function. Agni governs metabolism. It is responsible for maintaining nutrition in the body and keeping the immune system in shape to battle diseases. Agni also helps to fight bacteria and toxins thus giving vitality and life to an individual. When one has his agni in perfect condition, a longer lifespan is expected, but when impaired, diseases start coming in and finally, when the agni fire is extinguished, death may be the result.

Taste and emotions One should be aware that there is a close relation between the food that one craves for and his emotions. Nowadays, terms like stress eating, emotional eating, over-eating etc have become much more like a norm. This should not be the case if one aims to be healthy. When a certain 'craving' is experienced, it is best to be aware that it might be one's emotions that are being suppressed. For example, pungent – hatred, sour – envy, sweet – attachment or love, bitter - grief, salty – greed and sour – envy. Being aware of this taste and emotion relation can be considered a secret to health as it makes a person understand himself better and gives him the opportunity to have healthier options.

Chapter 16: Annar (Pomeground).

Just in case you first learn about pomegranates: Pomegranates are the orange-sized fruits with a healthy ruby-red outer skin and sweet arils-a red gelatinous flesh that contains lots of seeds. The pomegranate seeds are nutritious and completely good, despite the many beliefs. Besides, every part of the grenade has health benefits-even the skin is used in dietary supplements as it is an excellent source of polyphenols, including condensed tannins, catechins, and prodelphinidins.

Pomegranates were identified in the early Bronze Age, and a dry grenade was found in the tomb of Thoth, one of the Ancient Egyptian deities, which makes us think that grenades were more common in the ancient times than they are now.

Pomegranate belongs to a superfood group, which means they are rich in nutrients that can protect every part of your wellbeing. They are packed with fiber, protein, omega-6 fatty acids, calcium, copper, selenium, potassium, magnesium, iron, zinc, phosphorus, and vitamins C, K, B6, and E. Pomegranate are a significant source of riboflavin, thiamine, niacin, folate, and choline as well. Flavonoids present in both the fruit of Pomegranate and its outer skin lead to improved health of the entire body. Pomegranates are low in saturated fat, cholesterol, and sodium, as well as having a relatively small glycemic index, meaning they don't cause a substantial increase in blood sugar.

Best Pomegranate safety benefits

The research never stays quiet and continues to discover new superfoods day after day. Fortunately, many researchers around the world have been paying attention to pomegranates, and also shocked by what they have already seen. It turns out that pomegranates will encourage not only better health but also a longer life. Particularly pomegranate juice has been shown to control blood sugar, improve heart health, and counter the inflammation of the whole body. Look at the top health benefits researchers have found for granaries:

Foster the safety of the heart and arteries.

A significant number of research and tests were carried out to investigate the pomegranates' heart-healthy benefits. Regular drinking of a pomegranate juice helps to reduce plaque, lower high blood pressure, and avoid inflammation and oxidation. The study was conducted with 10 patients who had consumed 1 and 3 years of pomegranate juice.

In another report, 13 men aged 39-68 who had high blood pressure drank 5 ounces of grenade juice, and their overall high blood pressure decreased by 7 percent after 6 hours. Besides, the experiment has shown that the intake of pomegranate juice enhances artery function.

Combatting chronic inflammation

It has been shown that Pomegranates decrease inflammatory activity in colon cancer and breast cancer cells-all thanks to the punicalagin present in the fruit. Pomegranate juice can also help prevent and treat chronic inflammation, which contributes mostly to severe diseases, including cancer, Alzheimer's disease, heart disease, and type 2 diabetes.

Strengthening sexual health.

Pomegranates have been acknowledged as a natural aphrodisiac for many years, and have also been connected with growth and fertility. Of course, scientists couldn't forget this fact, and they have already undertaken a host of studies showing that Pomegranate's production encourages sexual health.

www.ingramcontent.com/pod-product-compliance
Lightning Source LLC
Chambersburg PA
CBHW071454070526
44578CB00001B/334